7 Costly Mistakes Health and Fitness Professionals Make And How to Avoid Them

Dr. Eric Cobb

NOTICE OF COPYRIGHT & MEDICAL DISCLAIMER

Copyright © 2014 by Z-Health® Performance Solutions, LLC

Published and distributed in the United States by:

Z-Health® Performance Solutions, LLC 8380 S. Kyrene Road, Suite 101 Tempe, AZ 85284 www.zhealtheducation.com

All rights reserved. No part of this book may be reproduced by any means or in any form whatsoever, nor may it be stored in a retrieval system, transmitted or otherwise copied for public or private use – other than as referenced material in articles and/or reviews - without the written permission of the author.

1ST Edition March 2014
2nd Edition July 2014

DISCLAIMER

The information provided by Z-Health Performance Solutions, LLC ("Z-Health") is strictly intended for your general knowledge and for informational purposes only.

The information contained in this or any Z-Health material, publications, or website (collectively "Z-Health Products") is not to be construed as medical recommendations, medical advice, diagnosis, treatment or as professional advice, nor is it intended for use as a substitute for consultation with or advice given by a medical practitioner, health care practitioner, or fitness professional. Before beginning this or any exercise or nutritional program, you should consult with your physician.

Neither Z-Health, its affiliates, agents nor any other party involved in the preparation, publication or distribution of the works presented herein is responsible for any errors or omissions in information provided in this or any Z-Health Product.

Z-Health makes no representation and assumes no responsibility for the accuracy of information contained herein or in any Z-Health Product. Z-Health specifically disclaims all responsibility and shall not be responsible for any liability, loss or risk, injury, damage, personal or otherwise, which is incurred as a consequence, directly or indirectly, of the use or application of any of the material contained in this product or any Z-Health Product.

Z-Health does not recommend, endorse or make any representation about the efficacy, appropriateness or suitability of any specific tests, products, procedures, treatments, services, opinions, health care providers or other information that may be contained on or available through this product any Z-Health Product.

Z-Health shall not be responsible or liable for the content, use, information, or products and services of these resources. Additionally, Z-Health shall not be held responsible for the conduct of any company, website or individual mentioned in this product, associated websites, or any Z-Health Product.

You are encouraged to confirm any information obtained from or through this product or any Z-Health Product with other sources, and review all information regarding any medical condition or treatment with your physician. Should you have any healthcare-related questions, please call or see your physician or other healthcare provider immediately.

You should never disregard medical advice or delay in seeking it because of something you have read here or in any Z-Health Products. The opinions expressed in this publication represent the views of Z-Health Performance Solutions, LLC.

If you have questions, please contact: info@zhealth.net.

Table of Contents

Special Note	1
Introduction	2
Costly Mistake #1	5
Costly Mistake #2	12
Costly Mistake #3	16
Costly Mistake #4	22
Costly Mistake #5	30
Costly Mistake #6	35
Costly Mistake #7	39
The Number One Thing	40
Programs versus People	41
Ignoring the Brain	42
Neural Hierarchy	43
Exercise Can Be Screwed Up	44
Quality Counts	45
Placing Blame	45
Are You Bored?	46
Results Matter	47
Client Retention	48
Magic Formula for a Dream Business	49
Accessing the Video and Audio	49

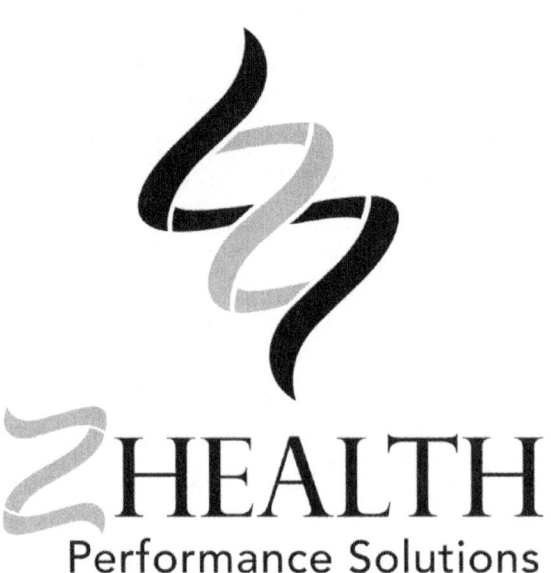

Special Note

The 7 Costly Mistakes that I share here were originally shared on a video, which was intended to be a product for sale on our website. After a number of Z-Health trainers found out about the product they urged me to reconsider and make it more widely available and accessible to personal trainers and other health and fitness professionals.

The best way to do that was to take the product that I already shot, have it transcribed, and made available for purchase. We have made every effort to edit the transcription and to keep the message and context intact.

If you scroll to the end, then you will see a link to a private web page where you can access the original video and audio files at no additional cost. I am making them available because I know that not everyone is a reader; some of you would rather enjoy watching a video or listening to just the audio. The private web page is there for you as a purchaser of this book. Enjoy!

Introduction

Hi, I am Dr. Eric Cobb, and for the next few minutes I am going to take off my doctor hat, and I am going to talk to you as a human being and a business person. I have been involved in the health and fitness business for over 20 years, and I am a coaches' coach. I find it incredibly frustrating to see people come and go in this industry. Looking at some statistics from just yesterday, 80% of personal trainers leave the industry within one year.

The career lifespan for a massage therapist is about 7 years. For chiropractors, it is about 12 year. It is very frustrating to me to see people in the helping professions becoming burned out so quickly or becoming injured so quickly.

I am going to spend some time sharing with you the most common mistakes that I have seen. These are things that go wrong, and they are going to seem very simple, but what is very important to me is that you understand that doing this stuff well is the world's greatest privilege.

It is a privilege to help people get out of pain, to rehabilitate them from injury, and to help them to achieve levels of physical performance that they have never achieved before. Really, it is a thing of beauty when you get to do it and you do it well.

The problem is how we approach this task. Most of us do not approach our profession like an elite athlete approaches his sport, and people go through this process of what is called habituation. This is when they get into their job, they are there for maybe a year or two years, and they begin to get comfortable. Whenever you get comfortable, you begin to forget two important things; education and communication.

Therefore, what I see in this field over and over is that people are in their businesses, they are talking the same way, and they are reading the same magazines over and over again. From these habits, they begin to be habituated into a certain style of working with the human body and speaking to their clients. Over time, it begins to cost them in terms of results and client retention.

Let's look at an elite athlete, for example an elite boxer. A boxer who has just won the world championship throws the same number and types of punches that an amateur boxer throws. The difference is that they have done it thousands more times and, most importantly, they have actually broken it down, and they have analyzed those punches to the smallest degree. And, they have had a coach do the same thing for them.

Whenever you want to be great at something, it's hard work. Being a great body professional, being a great personal trainer, chiropractor, massage therapist, physical therapist, or medical physician is difficult. If you want to be the best, then it requires work.

Therefore, I am going to share with you the common mistakes that people make as well as give you some strategies to avoid them. I want to give you a leap across your competition as well as save you a bunch of years of making mistakes so that your business can take on the structure that you originally wanted it to have in order to give you the life that you are looking to lead.

Let's get started.

Costly Mistake #1

In the introduction, I mentioned what I call the three "shun" sisters. The three shun sisters are education, communication, and habituation. These are things that we have to learn to deal with if we want to really excel in our given profession.

I mentioned before that helping people to get out of pain might be the best gift that you can ever give them, but then I stated that being able to take them from pain to performance, that is something that can revolutionize their life and yours in the same time frame.

It is an amazing thing to be able to do. Whenever I was first in practice, I had this realization. I was really frustrated when I was a young doctor because I was in practice and people kept coming to me about pain issues. Every morning I got up, and I put on this metaphorical big blow up suit that had Advil written across it.

I had this morning ritual because I thought that I was just a walking Advil. People came into my office and said, "Hey, my neck hurts. My back hurts." And after a couple of years of that, I got really frustrated.

Then something interesting happened, and this was part of that education for me. I was in my office and a woman came in. She had two kids with her, and I could hear her screaming at her kids in the parking lot. I mean seriously screaming. Not to the point that I needed to call Child Protective Services or anything, but it was weird. It was really intense and she came in and she was still yelling at her kids. After hearing this I finished up with my previous patient and I went out immediately grabbed her.

I said, "Hey, come on back. Let's get you back into the treatment room." And so, we went back. I started talking with her and I said, "What's going on?" and she said, "Oh, my head's killing me. It's been killing me for the last three days." So, I worked with her. It was a typical session. I was able to get her headache to go away in about 3-4 minutes, and then I just kept her there so that she could relax.

After less than 20 minutes, we were done. She walked out of my office, and the very first thing that she did is she went to the chair where her kids were sitting. She knelt down in front of them. She put her arm around both of them. She hugged them and apologized for her behavior.

It was in that moment that I had a big epiphany. I learned that sometimes the best gift that I can give people is getting them out of pain. Maybe it was not talking to them about their diet today. Maybe it was not dealing with their desire to win the golf championship today.

Sometimes, helping people to get out of pain is the biggest gift that I can give them and their families. That put me on a search to be good at that. Since that day I have had similar experiences though not just in pain but also in performance.

First and foremost, if you are going to be a pro in any industry, then you have to continue your educational process throughout your career. It is so easy to become habituated. That is how our brain works.

What I am going to talk about a little bit later are the different aspects of neurophysiology because that is the stuff that no one is talking about in our industry yet, not in a really practical way.

We get buzzwords that come around. People talk about the brain, neuro-fitness, and all that stuff. We have been researching and turning that research into practical information for 15 plus years. I am going to give you some real nuggets that you can begin to use immediately.

What is most fascinating in studying the brain is how it affects our ability to help people to get out of pain and to improve their lives, improve their sports performance, and improve their function at work. Studying the brain teaches us all about communicating with people.

The first thing that I really want to get into today is the idea of becoming a better businessperson by being a better listener. I was reading this great book, and it is by a guy that specializes in teaching other people how to talk to their family and their loved ones. He is a psychologist and he was a hostage negotiator. He trains hostage negotiation teams, and he has this unique quote, which was based on the experiences that he had.

He said that when he was in school he had a great professor who was really well respected. This professor had been watching him throughout a couple of his courses, and at one point he calls him over and he says, "Hey, you know, I have a suggestion for you."

He said, "I think you could be really, really good at this whole helping people skill set, but you have to learn one really important thing." And the guy that wrote the book, he said, "Well, what's that?" and his professor said, "You need to learn how to be more interested than interesting." The first time that I read that, I thought, "Wow. That is profound."

Walk into any gym or any doctor's office around the country and more often than not, you are going to see the professional trying to be more interesting than interested. What that means at the most basic level is that human beings, when they walk into your business, want to connect with you. They want to know that they can trust you; that they can talk to you. Whoever you are, if you spend the majority of your time talking to people rather than listening to them, then you are making one of the gravest errors that you can make in your business.

So, are there skills that you can develop to help this? Absolutely. Communication is something that can be studied. There are a tremendous number of great books available. You can look at our website. If you look at our website, we have a reading section that you can go to. Click Here

In there, you are going to see a number of books that we recommend on learning how to talk to people. It is one of those strange skill sets because most of our lives we have been talking to people. We learned to speak when we were really young. You figured out, that when you made this cool sound, your mom came over and gave you something to eat. We are pretty hooked on the whole communication thing.

The problem is that we get into a habituated position with it. For example, once we are in a high school, we already think that we know how to talk to people. Moreover, I can distinctly remember thinking this when I was a young man. I was meeting with a guy who was a school counselor, and we were talking about getting into graduate school and having an interview. We were having this conversation when he said, "Well, how do you think you can communicate your ideas to the person you are going to be interviewing?" and I said, "Well, I think I am a really good communicator." Then, he looked at me and he laughed.

He said, "Yeah, I thought I was too when I was 20." I kind of got offended and I thought, "Well, what do you mean?" and he said, "Listen," he said, "I've been studying communication my whole life and the older I get and the more I study and the more I realize, it's not just about thinking and reading about communication. It's about practicing it."

So, one of the things that I am going to tell you is this. In terms of strategy, tomorrow, when you walk into your place of business or you walk into your own home and you begin talking to people that actually do matter to you, you should give yourself 5 seconds whenever they start speaking, and then closely watch your own response.

One of the most common things that we do whenever people begin giving us information is called a writing reflex. The writing reflex basically is our immediate response that wants to tell them exactly what they need to do to fix their problem.

Most people communicate in that style and in that fashion. Think about how you talk to your children, how you talk to your spouse, and how you talk to your clients. You might hear someone say, "Hey man, my shoulder hurts." On the other hand, you might hear someone say, "I was watching you work out yesterday and you did this stupid exercise. You need to quit." Whenever we communicate in that style, it actually creates a tremendous amount of resistance, and that really starts to put it back into the, "Hey, listen to me," category rather than, "I am listening to you" category.

So for now, what I want you to remember is that phrase, "I am listening to you." If you really want to build your business, beyond leaps and bounds, and if you want to improve your relationships in ways that you never would have imagined possible, then you should begin working on becoming **more interested than interesting.**

Costly Mistake #2

We are now going to talk about one of my favorite topics that I speak about all the time for fitness and health care professionals. When someone walks into your office and they sit down in front of you, it is very tempting to go back to a book or a magazine and say, "Alright, here is your program, here is what you need." However, the mistake that people make, the number one mistake, is this. We trust programs or we give programs rather than just looking at and working with people. We value programs over people, and that is a huge mistake because the human body is not simple.

In fact, it is the most complicated and mysterious thing in the universe, in my opinion. After many years in the field of neuroscience, I have learned the value of looking at some research articles. Right now, 60,000 plus neuroscience articles are being published every year, and the very top scientists in this field are just scratching the surface.

There is so much to know. Unfortunately, what often happens is that when people walk through our door, we default to this idea that, "Hey, I got this perfect program for you." Whenever we have someone come in and we do our initial evaluation, we say, "If we do this for the next 12 weeks, then the end result is you should be happy." Very often, that flies in the face of what we are going to see if we just pay attention. **So, remember, you should never value programs over people.**

People do not work that way. We have too many different factors that can go wrong. Even though you may have on paper what you consider the perfect program, there will be someone that comes to you with a weight loss goal, and you should not tell him or her, "Okay, this is going to be the perfect weight-loss program for you based on my initial assessment. In the next 16 weeks I expect you to lose two pounds a week."

Instead, you should be more interested than interesting, and you should find out whether they are in the middle of divorce proceedings, or if they have just lost their job, or if their child has been diagnosed with leukemia, or if they have some other kind of life stressor that has recently happened.

That stress can result in this training program that you believe is the best training program ever written in the history of the planet actually makes them worse. It is too stressful. It is too hard because the accumulative stress from their life is piling up on top of the stress that you are giving them. If you have never talked to them and you do not pay attention to that stuff, then you wind up confused and frustrated.

Now, we are 8 weeks in, and the client has not lost nearly as much weight and they are complaining and saying, "I don't understand. I'm not losing weight and in fact, I feel worse. My knees hurt or my shoulder's hurting. My back's hurting." If we look at things statistically, then this describes about 85% of the people that begin fitness programs.

Therefore, this is one of the huge mistakes that we see day in and day out. People come in and because of our education, we believe that if we follow a set pattern all the time with everyone, then we will get the results that the client wants. The fact is that you have to begin valuing what you see in them and what they say to you far more than you ever value anything that you put down on paper.

If you can do that, then you can learn the basic skill set of observation. You will begin paying attention and saying, "Man, you look really, really tired today. How do you feel?" If you see additional stress on their face, if you see that their breathing is becoming aberrant, or if you see that their posture is getting worse, then that is a good sign that they are not happy, or at least that their nervous system is under too much stress in your environment.

Therefore, as you begin to learn to notice those small cues, you can modify what you do on the fly, help them to reduce their stress, and help them to get the results that they want over time. So, remember that you have to **value your people over your programs**.

Costly Mistake #3

We have discussed a couple of very important topics thus far. Now, I am going to move into something that hopefully will begin to help you to revolutionize your thought process about how you look at people as well as how you work with people. For the last 20 years, I have been on a quest if you will. I do not like to use the term "adventure" because this has really been a passion of mine. Something that has driven me to get up early, to stay up late, to study and read constantly, to go through thousands upon thousands of books, magazine articles, training sessions, and attend courses. I do all of this because I am passionate about helping people to improve.

If you are involved in the helping professions, then you need to begin shifting your focus to the human brain. It is this beautiful, complex, and mysterious organ. The more that we study it, the more we learn about it. The more we learn, the more we are going to know about how to create the changes that our clients want from us and that we want for ourselves.

However, this is the unfortunate part of the lecture because talking about the brain seems so big and so nebulous that most people, whenever I begin to use terms like neuroscience, kind of just shut down, go blank, and become disinterested in the subject because they perceive that it is just too complicated. The fact is, this is not so complicated that you cannot make use of it; you must begin to understand it.

Whenever we work with people, we are constantly reminded of the fact that people are complex. They come in and they complain of a left knee pain, or they come in and say, "Do you know what? I have worked out off and on for the last 5 years. I can never seem to make any progress."

We normally blame them at that point in the back of our heads. We say, "Yeah, you probably just didn't know what you were doing or you didn't work hard enough just like everyone else." If you understand the brain, then you will begin to rethink that perspective because the fact is that the human brain is in charge of it all. Therefore, if you have a client that comes in and they want hypertrophy, then they want to get bigger, and they want to get stronger. **The target of your training is the brain whether you know it or not.**

Someone comes in with a stiff neck, and you are doing manipulation or mobilization, if that is your thing. You are doing some massage or you are giving exercises because that is what you do. All of that is still targeting the brain whether you know it or not. Therefore, if you are going to become an elite professional, or if you want to continue to increase the level of service that you provide, then you should **begin to understand how the brain functions; this is absolutely essential.**

Let me give you a classic example of why this is so important. Everybody that works with other human beings has people that come in and they complain of their problem area, whatever that is. They say, "Oh yeah, my right shoulder is bugging me again. Oh my back, I've got a bad back." I always ask them, "What did it do? Did it go out? Did you stay out late drinking? What did it do? Why is it a bad back?" I ask these questions because people need to think about what they are saying. There has to be a reason for the pain that they are experiencing. These things do not just occur unexpectedly.

So, one of the ways that this works is that modern neuroscience has really given us an understanding that whenever we are experiencing that bad back pain, or that shoulder pain, or that knee pain, it does not mean that the spot is hurt. It does not mean that there is an injury there. Someone is complaining about their shoulder, and most of us immediately rush to the conclusion that, "Oh, they've got a rotator cuff tear. They've got a biceps problem. They've got a labral tear. They've got," what I like to call, "Joint termites." We have all these crazy things that we say to them when in fact the experience of the pain is occurring in their brain, and it may be occurring for no reason associated with their shoulder.

The way that the brain functions is like this: Maybe early on in their life that person was a baseball pitcher, and maybe he did have an acute injury. Therefore, because of that acute injury, he had pain for 8 weeks.

Well, guess what, whenever we practice something, we get good at it. And so, if your brain has this really nicely developed pain pathway for your shoulder, then whenever something else is going wrong in your life, and your stress levels are up, your brain is just frustrated with you and it is saying, "Listen, you're violating everything that I want you to do." The brain will often revisit an old pain in order to make you change your behavior. It is important to realize that most of the time that is what we are really dealing with.

We are not dealing with people who are broken. We are dealing with people whose brain is trying to communicate to them in a way that will get their attention. Now, that may sound a little farfetched to you, but that is how complicated we are. One of the best things that you can begin to do in this process is to broaden your vision, broaden your horizon, and broaden your possibility list. People come in and they are going to complain about different things to you. It is important to give yourself permission to begin thinking this way, "Okay, they've got knee pain. That doesn't mean that their knee is messed up." It could be the case, but in most cases, it is probably not true. Instead, you should ask yourself the question, "What else could be going on?"

You have to learn how to evaluate people. You should make a habit of watching them move and noting their gait. As you begin to understand and explore this in greater depth, what you will quickly begin to see is that you have this capacity and skill to help get rid of all these different little aches and pains; you have the capacity and skill to remove performance blockages that people have had for years. You do this not by focusing on the same old area, but rather by doing something completely different. That is the huge value of learning to pay attention to neuroscience in what you do.

We have talked about the need to make sure that we are listening more. We have talked about the need to be interested more than the need to be interesting. We have talked about the need to value people over programs. In this particular case, it is really simple. **Quit ignoring the brain.** You should never think, "Ah, I just can't understand that stuff." We are actually harming ourselves, and we are harming our clients by thinking this. **Just begin to expand your thought possibilities beyond looking at just the area that they are complaining about.**

Costly Mistake #4

In our last section, I talked about the fact that we can no longer afford to ignore the brain in working with human beings. It is vital to me that you begin to understand that. Now, if I were to stop there, then I would be committing one of the gravest errors that you can commit in coaching. This is something that I have learned from a combative instructor that I trained with for years; he always uses the idea that you need to be a coach and not a critic because a critic can only tell you what is wrong. A coach is someone who can tell you what is wrong, and they have some ideas and drills to help you fix it.

I have told you that you should not ignore the brain. I am going to give you some more specifics about what that means as well as what you can do about it. In order to really understand the human brain and how it affects function and movement, you have to realize that it is an integrative system. I am going to give you some very simple examples. However, we need to look at our education. We have to study our communication, and we have to avoid habituation.

I became a neuromuscular skeletal expert only after spending close to a million dollars on my education and attending numerous specialized courses. It is not that I never created results following what I learned in my formal education. It is not that I did not make clients happy or my patients happy. It is not that the athletes that I worked with did not improve. However, there was always this nagging belief for me that, "Man, I think that I should be capable of doing more for them."

Now, I am speaking for most of the athletes that I have worked with by saying that it always seemed like there were barriers in place that I could never figure out how to break down. No matter how much soft tissue work, or how much stretching and strength training that I put into my clients, there were still some barriers that I could not break down. This was true regardless of everything else that I did in my early professional career. As that frustration grew, it was really one of the biggest blessings that I have ever had in my life because it drove me into this obsessive quest for what actually makes people better. When I began to look at the neuroscience, I found some really interesting things that became useful in breaking down those barriers.

Let me introduce this idea to you called the performance hierarchy. This is a term that I use, but it helps to really begin to narrow down our focus on what can go wrong in the human body as well as what we need to do about it. So, the performance hierarchy works like this. As I am moving through my life, my brain is in charge, number one, of keeping me alive, and the way that it keeps me alive is by making predictions about my immediate environment as well as what is about to happen.

Now, prediction is a high-level cognitive function, but it can only happen in an optimal fashion whenever we have three systems that are functioning at a high level. Those three systems, in order, are the visual system, the vestibular system, and the proprioceptive system. The vestibular system, if you are not familiar with it, is what most people call their inner ear, and it is in charge of balance. The somatosensory or proprioceptive system is the system that gives our joints and muscles the opportunity to send signals from the periphery nervous system into our spinal cord, and then up to our brain so that our brain knows what we are doing.

The quality of your movement and athletic performance, as well as the amount of pain that you have, and your skills and abilities will be determined by how well these systems operate independently and how well they integrate together.

Now, the way that we explain this to clients is simple. We tell them that your brain has a GPS because most people have at least seen one before; they can associate the brain's functions to those satellites that triangulate with the central unit. They can make the connection that because of those signals, your GPS is able to figure out where you are in space as well as where you are on the planet.

This is a perfect example of how the brain works because what is happening all the time is we have our three satellite systems. We have the visual system. We have the vestibular system. We have the proprioceptive system. All three of them are active all the time; they are sending signals into the brain, and the brain is kind of functioning like the GPS unit in your car.

It is integrating the information that is coming in and it is saying, "All right, based on the information I'm receiving, I'm currently in this location, moving at this speed, and I expect to reach my destination at this time." That is really how our brain works. Now, most of us have had the experience of a GPS going badly wrong. You are traveling in a big city, and you have the big, tall concrete skyscrapers beside you when you drive in. Sometimes, when you really need it, the GPS can lose its signal.

This is a bad thing because now your brain, which keeps you safe via prediction, has lost its signaling capability. For example, you may lose signaling from your ankle because you have had an ankle sprain. Now, because of the swelling from that ankle sprain, you are getting fewer signals, or you are receiving fewer signals that are useful signals from the ankle.

Then, because you did not really do any good rehab on it, you are 6 weeks into the injury, and scar tissue is beginning to build up. That scar tissue is now causing one of the joints to become tighter and tighter. As the joints closed up, the brain is getting some aberrant signals.

Therefore, not only am I losing signals, but also I may be getting some cross signaling, and now my brain is getting really confused. What the brain will begin to do is alter how I walk as well as how my foot strikes the ground. I am now going to get a cascading effect that will continue up to the rest of my body, which may cause issues somewhere else.

Therefore, whenever we evaluate any athlete or any client that we are working with, if you are going to be considered, an elite, true movement specialist, then you have to get some more education. You have to be able to evaluate the visual system. The visual system is complex; it is incredibly complex.

Nevertheless, you can learn some of the basics. You can learn how to test it, and you can learn how to give drills to improve it. You can test basic eye movements. You can figure out that the eyes converge and diverge because there are really only four basic categories of movement that the eyes need to do. If you learn a test from each one of them, then you can learn how to work with them.

Then, you need to be able to evaluate the vestibular system. Now, most people think, "Hey, I can do balance work with my clients." Well, when they think balance, what they normally think about is standing on some type of unstable surface, such as a bosu ball, foam roller, another athlete, a cat, or whatever you can step on that is somewhat wobbly.

These create a challenge, but in general, when people step on something unstable, they keep their heads still. However, if they keep their heads still, then they are actually violating one of the most important components of balance training.

They are violating a principle rule of balance training because your inner ear is designed to help you to figure out what is going on when your head is in motion, what is going on when you are moving forward, and what is going on when you are jumping up and down. You need to understand that there are really just two things that the vestibular system tells you from its constant analysis of your environment. The vestibular system is continually asking, "Which way am I going?" and "Which way is up?" If you understand that as well as the basic mechanics of its function, then you can design exercises that challenge it, stimulate it, and make it work better for you.

Then finally, we get into the proprioceptive system. Now, this is amazing stuff. Most of us are already doing a lot of proprioceptive work. If you help people to move, guess what, you are training the proprioceptive system. However, the types of questions that you should be asking are, "What type of signaling are you creating?" as well as "Are you giving them good satellite information or are you kind of giving them jumbled stuff?" If we look at how this system is built, then we realize that it needs precise information.

The way that we approach proprioceptive training in the Z-Health system is we ask, "Listen, what gives us the greatest amount of signaling?" We could go through a lot of complicated neurology, but from our perspective, the best thing that you can do to improve signaling from the body into the brain is to work on the joints.

Now, whenever we do joint-based work, we are not just exercising the joints. We are exercising the muscles, the ligaments, and even the skin that overlie the joints. These exercises are going to create a signaling pathway up into the brain that could be very useful or detrimental based on how you do it.

So, in the beginning, you have to have a system in place that says, "Hey, how are the joints in the foot moving? How are the joints in their thoracic spine moving? How are the joints in their neck moving? Do they have control of that area? Can they turn and twist? Can they laterally glide? Can they do that with every part of their body?" You need to do this type of questioning because if your clients cannot do these movements, then what that tells us is that there are some signaling issues. If we can fix that, then almost miraculous things can occur.

When we said, do not ignore the brain, we were saying that you have three major systems that you need to learn how to assess and work with **if you're going to really function as the most elite in your field. Those systems are the visual system, the vestibular system, and then the proprioceptive (somatosensory) system.** Whenever you begin to increase your education about these three systems, what you are going to create for your own body and for that of your clients will amaze you.

Costly Mistake #5

Alright now, we are to one of my favorite topics to discuss, which is this, **"Exercise is not so simple that you can't screw it up."** That is something that you really should write down, put quotes on it, and put it up on your wall.

So, let me set it up for you. Researchers in Finland took 229 people, and they conducted a study on exercise science. It was a very well controlled study. They took 229 people, and they put them on a 17-week combined cardio and strength-training program, which was comparable to the environment that you would find in any gym around the world. I make this assertion because people come in and we want to do what is good for them. We want to help them. We want to improve their cardiovascular fitness. We want to improve their strength.

In this study, they did pre-training testing. They did one rep max testing. They did different VO2 max as well as other cardiac indicator testing, and then they put them through the standardized 17-week training program.

After 17 weeks, one third of the group was classified as high responders. They did really, really well. Over the 17 weeks, their strength improved. Their cardiovascular fitness improved, and the improvement was in the 30-40% range.

After 17 weeks, 30-40% improvement is okay. It is not earth shattering but it is pretty good. There was also a group considered the normal responders. The normal responders averaged somewhere between 10% to 18% improvement in their tests after 17 weeks. So basically, they were getting 1% improvement in fitness or strength each week that they were training.

Now personally, I am not that excited about those results. I do not want to come up to someone and say that I am only interested in getting him or her 1% better each week. Now, if I were already an elite athlete, then yes 1% per week would make you amazing. However, most people that we are seeing or working with are not elite athletes.

So anyway, that was the middle group. Then, we get into the really interesting stuff because the bottom part of the study had people that were not just low responders, they were in fact labeled as non-responders because their average rate of improvement over the course of 17 weeks in the combined strength and cardio training program was an astonishing -8%.

I want you to stop and just let that sink in, -8%. Think about that. Seventeen weeks of hard work to get slower, fatter, and less fit. That's fantastic. You know people are going to be knocking down my door right now to sign up for that program, right? That sounds great. I can give you 4 hours a week to get weaker.

Now, what was weird about this was the scientist that ran the study repeated it, and then repeated it again, and then repeated it again. They got the same results over time consistently in these different studies. This was due to a glaring logical error that was made, and it is very frustrating to me.

They said, "Wow, we're getting this consistent group of people who seem to not respond to exercise." Moreover, by doing what all good scientists do, they came up with the theory and labeled them "genetic non-responders to exercise." Again, let that one just sink in.

Imagine that a baby is born 20 years from now, and we get to do a DNA test on them. Therefore, as soon as they are able to understand language, we say, "Child, I'm very sorry. You are a genetic non-responder to exercise. You are destined to be fat, weak, and slow." This is just a strange idea to me. The assumption that the scientist had to make was that exercise is so simple that you cannot screw it up. Think about that.

However, nowhere in any of these studies did they have someone there videotaping the client, and going, "That is bad form on the bench press." There was no one filming them doing their cardio work going, "Man, he's going into a really stressed state, you can see it on his face. We need to back him off a little bit because if he keeps pushing at that intensity for the next 17 weeks, then he's actually going to wear himself out." They had this issue because they thought that exercise is just exercise. Those Finnish researchers believed that anyone could do it.

I want to give you a different perspective. In pharmacology, there is this great term called the MED, the Minimal Effective Dose. If you have a condition, you see a physician. The physician prescribes the correct drug for you. You go to the pharmacist, you fill the prescription, and you need to take that drug at the right dose because if you take too little of it, then it may not have any impact on the symptoms or condition that you currently have.

You could take the right dose. You may feel better, and then if you take an excessive amount, guess what? It may kill you. Well, exercise is a drug. You have to begin by thinking of it that way.

Exercise includes rehabilitative exercise, gym exercise, and sport training exercise. They are all drugs. So, as an elite professional, what I have to understand is that I am kind of like the pharmacist to some degree. I have to figure out how much exercise to prescribe to my patient based on a whole lot of other stuff that is going on with them. I also have to determine if it is even possible for me to administer the correct dose of exercise to my patient because when I give them the wrong dose there are two things that could potentially happen; either nothing happens or bad things happen. If I exercise you too little, then I do not challenge your body. Conversely, if I exercise you too much, then I could threaten your body enough to create an adaptation to the "drug."

However, that is generally not something that we see in the industry. What we see instead is the phenomenon of constant overdosing because people have begun to believe in hard work versus smart work. If we know anything from the study that I am discussing right now, then we know that if we do the wrong thing, we can screw the exercise regimen up. It is not that easy. Therefore, our job as an elite professional is to begin to understand the signs of overstressing people as well as the signs of under stressing people, and that is something that you can develop in many different ways.

So remember, **the Minimal Effective Dose (MED) of exercise is the crucial skill set that you need to develop as an elite professional** to help your clients to reach the body of their dreams as well as to help you to get the business that you have always wanted.

Costly Mistake #6

We are now to one of my favorite topics to discuss, and this topic is quality. Now, if you think back to the idea that exercise is not so simple that you can't screw it up, I talked about the idea that we have to view exercise as a drug, right? Remember that we said that there is a minimal effective dose of a drug, and if we give you too little of it, then it does not work. If we give you the right amount, then we will probably get what we are looking for. If we give you too much, then all kinds of bad things can happen, called effects, or it could even kill you.

Now, imagine what would happen if I gave you a contaminated drug. If it was the right drug, then I could expect these good things to occur. I give you a good drug at the right dosage, and excellent stuff happens. **Well, the problem is that in exercise, the quality of the substance is the quality of the repetition that is performed by the athlete.** So, when someone comes in and they are doing a bench press, **whenever they do a lousy bench press, that is like getting a contaminated drug.** We cannot trust the results.

I might give you too little. I might give you too much. So man, things get really, really confusing, and this is one of the industry standards that I find most frustrating. Industry standards kind of work like this: If you pick up any training article, it is going to talk about the perfect set rep as well as the perfect tempo scheme.

You are going to have constant arguments by professionals that are going to say something to the effect of, "I think four sets of eight are better than eight sets of four." And, part of your brain has to go, "Huh?" because overtime, there are only so many variables or so many ways that we can mess around with the numbers. However, if we take a step back, and we look at everyone else around us, then we realize that every other industry is based on accuracy and quality, right?

One of the examples that I often use is this: let us assume that your business is booming, and you are going to hire a new receptionist. Someone comes in for an interview, and you are sit down with them and say, "Okay, tell me about your typing skills." And they go, "I type 300 words a minute." Part of your brain has to say, "Holy cow, 300 words a minute. I have got to see this." You sit here, you sit him down, and he just goes tearing across the keyboard. At the end of this demonstration, you go, "Okay, hit print. I have got to see this." They hit print and the paper comes out, and you have 300 words, but they are not really words. They are just jumbled letters and you ask, "What the heck?" and they say, "Well, I know people like fast typists."

The point is not the speed. The point is speed with accuracy. Therefore, we have to think about exercise the same way. I do not care how many sets and reps you can do. I care about the quality of every single rep that you perform because if you mess that up, then the end result will never be what you are hoping for.. As an exercise professional and as a rehab professional, if you are going to move into the elite category or if you are already in that elite trainer category, then we have to have a near obsession with knowing the perfect form of every exercise as well as emphasizing it every single time. That is our job.

It is interesting to me because I see trainers getting bored in training sessions. I do not know how you could be bored. There is so much stuff to pay attention to during the session. Someone sits down to do an exercise, and you are not just watching them pick up the bar or whatever. Instead, you are looking at their feet, and then you are looking at their knees and their hips as well as the alignment of their spine. You are assessing their posture by asking yourself a series of questions, such as "Does she have too much tension in her face?" That is a lot of stuff to keep track of at once. However, every single one of those elements is a part of ensuring good rep quality.

This a hallmark difference between the amateur and the pro in our professions, and whenever I talk about repetition, some people go, "Well, that doesn't really apply to my arena." Ah, it absolutely does. If you are a running coach, swimming coach, baseball coach, or tennis coach, then every single technique of every sport can be broken down into a component part called the repetition. It is your job as an elite trainer to look at each component and go, "Is that a perfect one?" because if it is not perfect, then ultimately, if I let that person practice imperfectly over time, then the end result is going to be compromised.

Remember, quality counts and it has to be your near obsession. When that becomes a part of who you are, then the results that you are going to achieve for yourself and for your clients are going to stagger you.

Costly Mistake #7

When things are going wrong in our businesses, we can point fingers in a couple of different directions. We can point them out and we can point them in. However, you have probably seen that old thing when I am pointing at you I have three more fingers that are pointing back at me.

In the fitness world and in the health care world this is right on. It is common that we blame our clients for their lack of results. We accuse them of not working hard. We accuse them of not following their diet. We accuse them of all these things, but at some point, we have to take a step back and as an elite professional ask, "Whose job is it to teach them? Whose job is it to help them to make the changes?" You have to make the fundamental realization that they are paying you, and that they have the right to expect exceptional service as your clients. Whenever your clients are not achieving their results, then that is something that should cause you to take a step back and ask, "Am I being as good as I can possibly be at my job?"

The Number One Thing

Think about the stuff that we have already discussed. We have talked about the number one thing that you have to do, which is that you have to learn to be more interested than interesting. You need to learn to listen, and you need to pay attention during every training session. I know that some times it drives you crazy to be an active listener, but it is necessary to do so.

In my practice years ago, I actually had a system in place to ensure this. The system was that my secretary knew all of my patients, and she knew the ones that caused an immediate response to seeing them on the schedule. We called them the "Oh no" patients, and we had a little initial for them because they were the people that were really hard for me to deal with. We all have clients like that, but we cannot blame them. If we remember to stop talking, and if we remember to stop telling them what to do and listen, i.e. if we become more interested than interesting, then those attitudes can begin to change. You will see a decline in your "Oh no" patients, and you will make a positive impact on their lives.

Programs versus People

After we talked about that, we started talking about the idea that we must learn to value people over programs. Most of us have experienced an environment where the mantra is, "Hey, you know what, the program is the thing." However, you need to ignore this mantra, and instead you should give clients an individualized strength program, an individualized hypertrophy program, or an individualized endurance training program for whatever their needs are rather than putting them through a generic program.

The fact is that I can have the best program in the world, but if it is applied to the wrong person, then it can destroy them. That is something that we absolutely have to learn to avoid. We have to pay attention to our clients all of the time.

Ignoring the Brain

Next, we talked about ignoring the brain. If you ignore the brain, then you are making the biggest mistake in your educational and professional life that you can ever make. We have learned over the last 20 years that the target of everything that we do with human beings is their brain. Whether they are trying to become stronger, more flexible, faster, get out of pain, or learn to read better. It does not matter. Everything is targeting the brain, so we have to understand how it works. We have to understand how it functions.

Neural Hierarchy

I then shared with you a really basic concept called the performance hierarchy and the neural GPS. The idea that we have a map in our brain as well as the idea that we have a map that is telling us where we are located in our physical environment is fundamental to our understanding of the human brain. This neural GPS tell us where we are going as well as how we are getting there.

If the information is lost, or if we lose the signal, or if we have bad signals coming in, then it causes a predictive problem for the brain that can cause all kinds of issues from pain to strength deficits, to range of motion and performance issues. We have to realize that both the GPS and the signals are important, and we have to learn to evaluate them and to train them if we want the best for our clients and for ourselves.

Exercise Can Be Screwed Up

Next, we talked about the scientific research into the fact that exercise is not as simple as most people would like us to believe, even the scientists. Remember that you can screw up any exercise regimen. Moreover, when you screw it up, then people not only do not get results, but you can also make them worse in the long-term.

We said that exercise is a drug, and just like with any other drug, you can receive an insufficient dose, or you can receive an overdose. I have to find the sweet spot when administering any drug, and there are ways to learn to assess people so that we can know that we are doing the right thing for them literally every single time that we see them. This is the idea that quality counts.

Quality Counts

If you look at a client that comes into your office, and you tell them that you want to see this amazing transformation week after week, then you need to realize that transformation will be built one repetition at a time. If the quality of the repetition is poor, then the quality of the end result cannot be anything but poor. It just does not work any other way. Therefore, we have to remind ourselves that quality counts.

Placing Blame

It is very easy to see that when we ignore issues we begin to place blame where it really does not belong. When a client comes in the door, they do not know what an exercise is supposed to look like. And more importantly, if their neural GPS is messed up and you are trying to teach them to do a bench press, then they might not even be able to understand the fact that they are doing it with more emphasis on the right arm, or that they are rotating because their movement maps are messed up.

It is so important that you understand each one of these categories because it will make you far less likely to blame your client. And when you stop blaming them, then you can actually begin creating the results that they need.

There are so many factors that go into this. There is stuff that I have talked about already. However, there is more than that. You know, I run into trainers all the time that are jumping on the latest bandwagon in fitness, whether it is some weird gadget, or the shake weight, or whatever it is that people are interested in at any given time. But if you keep following trends, then there is a reason that you are doing it.

Are You Bored?

The reason that you are following trends is you are bored. Whenever you get bored, you get lost in all these other training modalities and ideas. We get bored because we are not actually paying attention in the first place to all the stuff that really matters.

With all of the different elements that can come into play, we have to understand that our business is built on three primary factors. The first factor, whether people like to admit it or not, is results. Results affect the vast majority of the people in the body professional industry, whether you are a personal trainer, a physical therapist, or a massage therapist.

Results Matter

People want results from you, and the fact is that most people do not get the results that they want and so they quit.

We live in a nation that has an underwhelming number of people exercising. If you read statistics, then 3% of the US population exercises regularly. In addition, 85% of people quit exercising within 6 weeks of beginning a program, and the majority of these quit because they are in pain or because they are injured, which is usually the result of someone not paying attention to all the stuff that we have been talking about. So, if you want to set yourself apart, then achieving results is the number one thing that you need to do.

Client Retention

Now, the beautiful part about being great at achieving the results safely and powerfully for your clients is that results lead you to the most important change element of all for your business, which is retention. People have asked me, "Doc, you know, if you could pick one thing to tell a fitness professional to really improve their business and to help their clients achieve everything they want to achieve, what does it need to be? Does it need to be a change in their strength training program, or a change in how they do cardio?"

And I respond, "No. The number one thing that you need to do is keep them. It is about retention because when I keep you long enough as a client by giving you progressive results over time, I educate you. I move out of this overbearing role to the role of mentor because I believe that every client that we see should be educated to the point where they can mostly take care of themselves. When we do that, we create this amazing environment from keeping these clients to them now bringing us new people, which we call referrals.

Magic Formula for a Dream Business

Therefore, results, retention, and referrals are really the magic formula for having the business of your dreams, which should lead to the life of your dreams as a body professional. The most elegant part of all of it for me is that it always begins with achieving results for the people that are paying for them. The most ethical thing that you can possibly do is to educate yourself, learn to communicate, and avoid habituating yourself to poor performance because when you do all of that stuff, you do the best for the people in your care as well as the best for yourself.

Good luck to you. I look forward to talking to you soon.

Accessing the Video and Audio

If you would rather access the audio and video, then go to:

http://www.zhealtheducation.com/7costlymistakes

Printed in Great Britain
by Amazon